Get to Know Your Buds™

Editing & Book Design:
    Shawn Aveningo Sanders
Cover Photograph (Bubba's Gift) / Design:
    Spurs Broken (aka Robert R. Sanders)
Get to Know Your Buds™ is a registered trademark
    in the state of Oregon, used with permission by
    Stage Two, Inc.
Printed in the United States of America.

Volume 3
ISBN-10: 0998099937
ISBN-13: 978-0-9980999-3-4

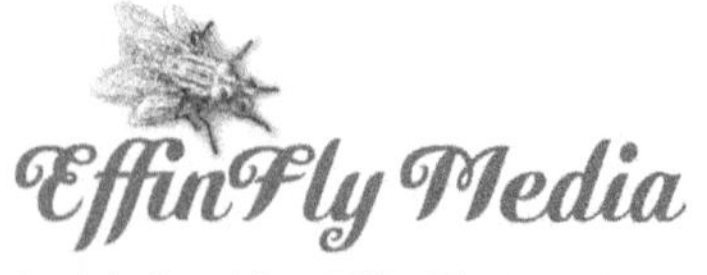

Published by EffinFly Media, 2017
Portland, Oregon
www.EffinFlyMedia.com

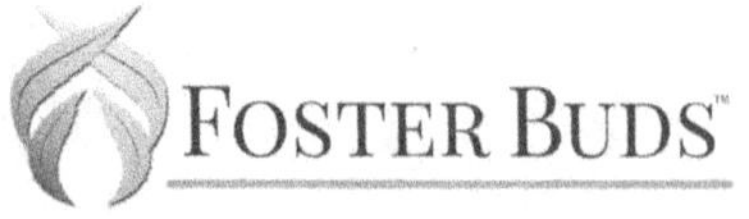

In partnership with Foster Buds™
(a Stage Two, Inc. Company)
www.FosterBuds.com

Get to Know Your Buds™

Personal Cannabis Journal

An EffinFly Media Publication

This Cannabis Journal
Belongs to:

____

Dated:

___ / ___ / ________

through

___ / ___ / ________

We hope you enjoy using this journal to *get to know your buds*. With hundreds of cannabis strains to choose from and new strains being crafted daily, remembering which ones are your favorites and which ones have been most effective for treating your ailments can be overwhelming.

That's why Foster Buds encourages cannabis users to keep track of what works for them personally. Whether you partake for pleasure or for medical reasons, this journal was created for you as a friendly, easy-to-use personal record to help foster good health, happiness and a better way of life.

Index of Entries

Strain/Product _______________________________

☐ Flower ☐ Extract ☐ Edible ☐ Topical

Dispensary _______________ Date _______

Grower _______________________________

☐Sativa ☐Indica ☐Hybrid (__%Sat __%Ind)

___%THC ___%CBD ___%CBN ___%CBG

Flavor/Aroma:

☐-Sweet ☐-Sour ☐-Citrus ☐-Berry

☐-Skunky ☐-Cheese ☐-Menthol

☐-Smokey ☐-Coffee ☐-Earthy

General Effects:

☐-Calming ☐-Couch Lock ☐-Sleepy

☐-Euphoric ☐-Mellow ☐-Creative

☐-Energetic ☐-Focused ☐-Munchies

Negative Effects:

☐-Dizzy ☐-Dry Mouth ☐-Headache

☐-Paranoid ☐-Vision ☐-Anxiety

Overall Rating: ☆ ☆ ☆ ☆ ☆

Notes..

Strain/Product _______________________

☐ Flower ☐ Extract ☐ Edible ☐ Topical

Dispensary _________________ Date _______

Grower ___________________________

☐Sativa ☐Indica ☐Hybrid (__%Sat __%Ind)

___%THC ___%CBD ___%CBN ___%CBG

Flavor/Aroma:

    ☐-Sweet ☐-Sour ☐-Citrus ☐-Berry

    ☐-Skunky ☐-Cheese ☐-Menthol

    ☐-Smokey ☐-Coffee ☐-Earthy

General Effects:

    ☐-Calming ☐-Couch Lock ☐-Sleepy

    ☐-Euphoric ☐-Mellow ☐-Creative

    ☐-Energetic ☐-Focused ☐-Munchies

Negative Effects:

    ☐-Dizzy ☐-Dry Mouth ☐-Headache

    ☐-Paranoid ☐-Vision ☐-Anxiety

Overall Rating: ☆ ☆ ☆ ☆ ☆

Notes...

Strain/Product ________________________________

☐ Flower ☐ Extract ☐ Edible ☐ Topical

Dispensary ___________________ Date _______

Grower ____________________________________

☐Sativa ☐Indica ☐Hybrid (__%Sat __%Ind)

___%THC ___%CBD ___%CBN ___%CBG

Flavor/Aroma:

☐-Sweet ☐-Sour ☐-Citrus ☐-Berry

☐-Skunky ☐-Cheese ☐-Menthol

☐-Smokey ☐-Coffee ☐-Earthy

General Effects:

☐-Calming ☐-Couch Lock ☐-Sleepy

☐-Euphoric ☐-Mellow ☐-Creative

☐-Energetic ☐-Focused ☐-Munchies

Negative Effects:

☐-Dizzy ☐-Dry Mouth ☐-Headache

☐-Paranoid ☐-Vision ☐-Anxiety

Overall Rating: ☆ ☆ ☆ ☆ ☆

Notes...

Strain/Product _______________________

☐ Flower ☐ Extract ☐ Edible ☐ Topical

Dispensary _________________ Date _______

Grower _____________________________

☐Sativa ☐Indica ☐Hybrid (__%Sat __%Ind)

___%THC ___%CBD ___%CBN ___%CBG

Flavor/Aroma:

    ☐-Sweet ☐-Sour ☐-Citrus ☐-Berry

    ☐-Skunky ☐-Cheese ☐-Menthol

    ☐-Smokey ☐-Coffee ☐-Earthy

General Effects:

    ☐-Calming ☐-Couch Lock ☐-Sleepy

    ☐-Euphoric ☐-Mellow ☐-Creative

    ☐-Energetic ☐-Focused ☐-Munchies

Negative Effects:

    ☐-Dizzy ☐-Dry Mouth ☐-Headache

    ☐-Paranoid ☐-Vision ☐-Anxiety

Overall Rating: ☆ ☆ ☆ ☆ ☆

Notes...

Strain/Product _______________________

☐ Flower ☐ Extract ☐ Edible ☐ Topical

Dispensary _________________ Date _______

Grower _______________________________

☐Sativa ☐Indica ☐Hybrid (__%Sat __%Ind)

___%THC ___%CBD ___%CBN ___%CBG

Flavor/Aroma:

☐-Sweet ☐-Sour ☐-Citrus ☐-Berry

☐-Skunky ☐-Cheese ☐-Menthol

☐-Smokey ☐-Coffee ☐-Earthy

General Effects:

☐-Calming ☐-Couch Lock ☐-Sleepy

☐-Euphoric ☐-Mellow ☐-Creative

☐-Energetic ☐-Focused ☐-Munchies

Negative Effects:

☐-Dizzy ☐-Dry Mouth ☐-Headache

☐-Paranoid ☐-Vision ☐-Anxiety

Overall Rating: ☆ ☆ ☆ ☆ ☆

Notes..

Strain/Product _______________________

☐ Flower ☐ Extract ☐ Edible ☐ Topical

Dispensary __________________ Date ______

Grower ______________________________

☐Sativa ☐Indica ☐Hybrid (__%Sat __%Ind)

___%THC ___%CBD ___%CBN ___%CBG

Flavor/Aroma:

☐-Sweet ☐-Sour ☐-Citrus ☐-Berry

☐-Skunky ☐-Cheese ☐-Menthol

☐-Smokey ☐-Coffee ☐-Earthy

General Effects:

☐-Calming ☐-Couch Lock ☐-Sleepy

☐-Euphoric ☐-Mellow ☐-Creative

☐-Energetic ☐-Focused ☐-Munchies

Negative Effects:

☐-Dizzy ☐-Dry Mouth ☐-Headache

☐-Paranoid ☐-Vision ☐-Anxiety

Overall Rating: ☆ ☆ ☆ ☆ ☆

Notes..

....

....

....

....

....

....

....

....

....

....

....

Strain/Product _______________________

☐ Flower ☐ Extract ☐ Edible ☐ Topical

Dispensary _________________ Date _______

Grower ___________________________________

☐Sativa ☐Indica ☐Hybrid (__%Sat __%Ind)

___%THC ___%CBD ___%CBN ___%CBG

Flavor/Aroma:

☐-Sweet ☐-Sour ☐-Citrus ☐-Berry

☐-Skunky ☐-Cheese ☐-Menthol

☐-Smokey ☐-Coffee ☐-Earthy

General Effects:

☐-Calming ☐-Couch Lock ☐-Sleepy

☐-Euphoric ☐-Mellow ☐-Creative

☐-Energetic ☐-Focused ☐-Munchies

Negative Effects:

☐-Dizzy ☐-Dry Mouth ☐-Headache

☐-Paranoid ☐-Vision ☐-Anxiety

Overall Rating: ☆   ☆   ☆   ☆   ☆

Notes..

....

....

....

....

....

....

....

....

....

....

....

Strain/Product ____________________

☐ Flower ☐ Extract ☐ Edible ☐ Topical

Dispensary _______________ Date ______

Grower _________________________

☐Sativa ☐Indica ☐Hybrid (__%Sat __%Ind)

___%THC ___%CBD ___%CBN ___%CBG

Flavor/Aroma:

☐-Sweet ☐-Sour ☐-Citrus ☐-Berry

☐-Skunky ☐-Cheese ☐-Menthol

☐-Smokey ☐-Coffee ☐-Earthy

General Effects:

☐-Calming ☐-Couch Lock ☐-Sleepy

☐-Euphoric ☐-Mellow ☐-Creative

☐-Energetic ☐-Focused ☐-Munchies

Negative Effects:

☐-Dizzy ☐-Dry Mouth ☐-Headache

☐-Paranoid ☐-Vision ☐-Anxiety

Overall Rating: ☆ ☆ ☆ ☆ ☆

Notes..

....

....

....

....

....

....

....

....

....

....

....

Strain/Product _______________________

☐ Flower ☐ Extract ☐ Edible ☐ Topical

Dispensary _________________ Date _______

Grower _______________________________

☐Sativa ☐Indica ☐Hybrid (__%Sat __%Ind)

___%THC ___%CBD ___%CBN ___%CBG

Flavor/Aroma:

    ☐-Sweet ☐-Sour ☐-Citrus ☐-Berry

    ☐-Skunky ☐-Cheese ☐-Menthol

    ☐-Smokey ☐-Coffee ☐-Earthy

General Effects:

    ☐-Calming ☐-Couch Lock ☐-Sleepy

    ☐-Euphoric ☐-Mellow ☐-Creative

    ☐-Energetic ☐-Focused ☐-Munchies

Negative Effects:

    ☐-Dizzy ☐-Dry Mouth ☐-Headache

    ☐-Paranoid ☐-Vision ☐-Anxiety

Overall Rating: ☆ ☆ ☆ ☆ ☆

Notes...

Strain/Product __________________________

☐ Flower ☐ Extract ☐ Edible ☐ Topical

Dispensary _________________ Date _______

Grower _______________________________

☐Sativa ☐Indica ☐Hybrid (__%Sat __%Ind)

___%THC ___%CBD ___%CBN ___%CBG

Flavor/Aroma:

☐-Sweet   ☐-Sour   ☐-Citrus   ☐-Berry

☐-Skunky   ☐-Cheese   ☐-Menthol

☐-Smokey   ☐-Coffee   ☐-Earthy

General Effects:

☐-Calming   ☐-Couch Lock   ☐-Sleepy

☐-Euphoric   ☐-Mellow   ☐-Creative

☐-Energetic ☐-Focused   ☐-Munchies

Negative Effects:

☐-Dizzy   ☐-Dry Mouth   ☐-Headache

☐-Paranoid   ☐-Vision   ☐-Anxiety

Overall Rating: ☆ ☆ ☆ ☆ ☆

Notes..

Strain/Product _______________________________

☐ Flower ☐ Extract ☐ Edible ☐ Topical

Dispensary _______________ Date _______

Grower _______________________________

☐Sativa ☐Indica ☐Hybrid (__%Sat __%Ind)

___%THC ___%CBD ___%CBN ___%CBG

Flavor/Aroma:

   ☐-Sweet ☐-Sour ☐-Citrus ☐-Berry

   ☐-Skunky ☐-Cheese ☐-Menthol

   ☐-Smokey ☐-Coffee ☐-Earthy

General Effects:

   ☐-Calming ☐-Couch Lock ☐-Sleepy

   ☐-Euphoric ☐-Mellow ☐-Creative

   ☐-Energetic ☐-Focused ☐-Munchies

Negative Effects:

   ☐-Dizzy ☐-Dry Mouth ☐-Headache

   ☐-Paranoid ☐-Vision ☐-Anxiety

Overall Rating: ☆   ☆   ☆   ☆   ☆

Notes..

....

....

....

....

....

....

....

....

....

....

....

Strain/Product _______________________

☐ Flower ☐ Extract ☐ Edible ☐ Topical

Dispensary _________________ Date _______

Grower _____________________________

☐Sativa ☐Indica ☐Hybrid (__%Sat __%Ind)

___%THC ___%CBD ___%CBN ___%CBG

Flavor/Aroma:

☐-Sweet ☐-Sour ☐-Citrus ☐-Berry

☐-Skunky ☐-Cheese ☐-Menthol

☐-Smokey ☐-Coffee ☐-Earthy

General Effects:

☐-Calming ☐-Couch Lock ☐-Sleepy

☐-Euphoric ☐-Mellow ☐-Creative

☐-Energetic ☐-Focused ☐-Munchies

Negative Effects:

☐-Dizzy ☐-Dry Mouth ☐-Headache

☐-Paranoid ☐-Vision ☐-Anxiety

Overall Rating: ☆ ☆ ☆ ☆ ☆

Notes..

Strain/Product ______________________

☐ Flower ☐ Extract ☐ Edible ☐ Topical

Dispensary ________________ Date ______

Grower ________________________________

☐Sativa ☐Indica ☐Hybrid (__%Sat __%Ind)

___%THC ___%CBD ___%CBN ___%CBG

Flavor/Aroma:

☐-Sweet ☐-Sour ☐-Citrus ☐-Berry

☐-Skunky ☐-Cheese ☐-Menthol

☐-Smokey ☐-Coffee ☐-Earthy

General Effects:

☐-Calming ☐-Couch Lock ☐-Sleepy

☐-Euphoric ☐-Mellow ☐-Creative

☐-Energetic ☐-Focused ☐-Munchies

Negative Effects:

☐-Dizzy ☐-Dry Mouth ☐-Headache

☐-Paranoid ☐-Vision ☐-Anxiety

Overall Rating: ☆ ☆ ☆ ☆ ☆

Notes..

Strain/Product _______________________

☐ Flower ☐ Extract ☐ Edible ☐ Topical

Dispensary ___________________ Date _______

Grower _______________________________

☐Sativa ☐Indica ☐Hybrid (__%Sat __%Ind)

___%THC ___%CBD ___%CBN ___%CBG

Flavor/Aroma:

☐-Sweet ☐-Sour ☐-Citrus ☐-Berry

☐-Skunky ☐-Cheese ☐-Menthol

☐-Smokey ☐-Coffee ☐-Earthy

General Effects:

☐-Calming ☐-Couch Lock ☐-Sleepy

☐-Euphoric ☐-Mellow ☐-Creative

☐-Energetic ☐-Focused ☐-Munchies

Negative Effects:

☐-Dizzy ☐-Dry Mouth ☐-Headache

☐-Paranoid ☐-Vision ☐-Anxiety

Overall Rating: ☆ ☆ ☆ ☆ ☆

Notes..

Strain/Product _______________________

☐ Flower ☐ Extract ☐ Edible ☐ Topical

Dispensary _______________ Date _______

Grower ___________________________________

☐Sativa ☐Indica ☐Hybrid (__%Sat __%Ind)

___%THC ___%CBD ___%CBN ___%CBG

Flavor/Aroma:

   ☐-Sweet ☐-Sour ☐-Citrus ☐-Berry

   ☐-Skunky ☐-Cheese ☐-Menthol

   ☐-Smokey ☐-Coffee ☐-Earthy

General Effects:

   ☐-Calming ☐-Couch Lock ☐-Sleepy

   ☐-Euphoric ☐-Mellow ☐-Creative

   ☐-Energetic ☐-Focused ☐-Munchies

Negative Effects:

   ☐-Dizzy ☐-Dry Mouth ☐-Headache

   ☐-Paranoid ☐-Vision ☐-Anxiety

Overall Rating: ☆   ☆   ☆   ☆   ☆

Notes...

Strain/Product _________________________

☐ Flower ☐ Extract ☐ Edible ☐ Topical

Dispensary _________________ Date _______

Grower _______________________________

☐Sativa ☐Indica ☐Hybrid (__%Sat __%Ind)

___%THC ___%CBD ___%CBN ___%CBG

Flavor/Aroma:

    ☐-Sweet ☐-Sour ☐-Citrus ☐-Berry

    ☐-Skunky ☐-Cheese ☐-Menthol

    ☐-Smokey ☐-Coffee ☐-Earthy

General Effects:

    ☐-Calming ☐-Couch Lock ☐-Sleepy

    ☐-Euphoric ☐-Mellow ☐-Creative

    ☐-Energetic ☐-Focused ☐-Munchies

Negative Effects:

    ☐-Dizzy ☐-Dry Mouth ☐-Headache

    ☐-Paranoid ☐-Vision ☐-Anxiety

Overall Rating: ☆　☆　☆　☆　☆

Notes..

....

....

....

....

....

....

....

....

....

....

....

Strain/Product _______________________

☐ Flower ☐ Extract ☐ Edible ☐ Topical

Dispensary _________________ Date _______

Grower _________________________________

☐Sativa ☐Indica ☐Hybrid (__%Sat __%Ind)

___%THC ___%CBD ___%CBN ___%CBG

Flavor/Aroma:

    ☐-Sweet ☐-Sour ☐-Citrus ☐-Berry

    ☐-Skunky ☐-Cheese ☐-Menthol

    ☐-Smokey ☐-Coffee ☐-Earthy

General Effects:

    ☐-Calming ☐-Couch Lock ☐-Sleepy

    ☐-Euphoric ☐-Mellow ☐-Creative

    ☐-Energetic ☐-Focused ☐-Munchies

Negative Effects:

    ☐-Dizzy ☐-Dry Mouth ☐-Headache

    ☐-Paranoid ☐-Vision ☐-Anxiety

Overall Rating: ☆ ☆ ☆ ☆ ☆

Notes..

Strain/Product _______________________

☐ Flower ☐ Extract ☐ Edible ☐ Topical

Dispensary __________________ Date _______

Grower ___________________________________

☐Sativa ☐Indica ☐Hybrid (__%Sat __%Ind)

___%THC ___%CBD ___%CBN ___%CBG

Flavor/Aroma:

    ☐-Sweet ☐-Sour ☐-Citrus ☐-Berry

    ☐-Skunky ☐-Cheese ☐-Menthol

    ☐-Smokey ☐-Coffee ☐-Earthy

General Effects:

    ☐-Calming ☐-Couch Lock ☐-Sleepy

    ☐-Euphoric ☐-Mellow ☐-Creative

    ☐-Energetic ☐-Focused ☐-Munchies

Negative Effects:

    ☐-Dizzy ☐-Dry Mouth ☐-Headache

    ☐-Paranoid ☐-Vision ☐-Anxiety

Overall Rating: ☆ ☆ ☆ ☆ ☆

Notes..

Strain/Product _______________________

☐ Flower ☐ Extract ☐ Edible ☐ Topical

Dispensary _________________ Date _______

Grower _______________________________

☐Sativa ☐Indica ☐Hybrid (__%Sat __%Ind)

___%THC ___%CBD ___%CBN ___%CBG

Flavor/Aroma:

☐-Sweet ☐-Sour ☐-Citrus ☐-Berry

☐-Skunky ☐-Cheese ☐-Menthol

☐-Smokey ☐-Coffee ☐-Earthy

General Effects:

☐-Calming ☐-Couch Lock ☐-Sleepy

☐-Euphoric ☐-Mellow ☐-Creative

☐-Energetic ☐-Focused ☐-Munchies

Negative Effects:

☐-Dizzy ☐-Dry Mouth ☐-Headache

☐-Paranoid ☐-Vision ☐-Anxiety

Overall Rating: ☆ ☆ ☆ ☆ ☆

Notes..

Strain/Product _______________________

☐ Flower ☐ Extract ☐ Edible ☐ Topical

Dispensary _________________ Date _______

Grower _________________________________

☐Sativa ☐Indica ☐Hybrid (__%Sat __%Ind)

___%THC ___%CBD ___%CBN ___%CBG

Flavor/Aroma:

    ☐-Sweet ☐-Sour ☐-Citrus ☐-Berry

    ☐-Skunky ☐-Cheese ☐-Menthol

    ☐-Smokey ☐-Coffee ☐-Earthy

General Effects:

    ☐-Calming ☐-Couch Lock ☐-Sleepy

    ☐-Euphoric ☐-Mellow ☐-Creative

    ☐-Energetic ☐-Focused ☐-Munchies

Negative Effects:

    ☐-Dizzy ☐-Dry Mouth ☐-Headache

    ☐-Paranoid ☐-Vision ☐-Anxiety

  Get to Know Your Buds™

Overall Rating: ☆ ☆ ☆ ☆ ☆

Notes..